Contents

INTRODUCTION

When diet and nutrition experts talk about "sugary" foods, they mean foods that contain lots of added sugar—which is any type of caloric sweetener that's added to foods. (Artificial sweeteners, such as sucralose, are non-caloric.) Sugar provides energy (i.e., calories) but no additional nutritional value. A little sugar might be okay, but a lot of sugar leads to weight gain. So followers of a no sugar diet avoid added sugars to promote weight loss.

It's no secret that most Americans have a sweet tooth. The average adult consumes about 22 teaspoons of added sugar a day. And that's on

top of any naturally occurring sugars consumed

through fruit, grains, and milk products.

Excessive sugar consumption has been linked to:

- obesity

- diabetes

- heart disease

- increased inflammation in the body

- high cholesterol

- high blood pressure

By adopting a no-sugar diet, your risk for these

health conditions significantly decreases. Keeping

this in mind may help you stick with a new diet

plan.

Keep reading for tips on how to get started,

foods to look out for, sweet substitutes to try,

and more.

NO SUGAR DIET

While there's no official definition, a no sugar

diet typically cuts out added sugar while allowing

for natural sugar. Experts agree reducing added

sugar intake improves overall health, but clarify

that you don't have to completely eliminate all

added sugar for such benefits."

The problem with sugary foods is eating or

drinking too much of them as they are high in

calories but not usually nutritious. They don't

have enough vitamins and minerals to make up for all the extra sugar.

Some people believe high fructose corn syrup is worse for your health than regular sugar, but there isn't enough credible scientific evidence to back that claim. They're both made up of a similar combination of glucose and fructose, and both have the same effect on the body.

Since there are several forms and types of sugars, it helps to know what you're looking for. If you see any of these on an ingredients list, the food has added sugars:

- Sugar
- Brown sugar

- High fructose corn syrup

- Corn sugar

- Syrup

- Corn syrup

- Fructose

- Glucose

- Sucrose

- Raw sugar

- Turbinado sugar

- Honey

Look at the Nutrition Facts Label to determine how much added sugar is in each serving. It may be just a small amount, or it might be a lot.

Honey is a natural sugar because bees make it, whereas regular sugar is made from beets, corn, or sugar cane. But nutritionally, honey is about the same as sugar or high fructose corn syrup, so foods made with honey are still considered sugary. Technically, honey does contain some nutrients, but not enough to improve your diet.

HOW IT WORKS

To begin, try to limit your added sugar intake to 100 to 200 calories per day (a tablespoon of honey has about 60 calories and a tablespoon of sugar about 50). The USDA's dietary recommendations suggest that everyone should limit added sugar intake to 10 percent of calories or less (so, 200 if you're consuming about 2000 calories a day).1 Once you get there, you can work to reduce sugars even further.

Read labels and choose the products that have the least added sugar. You don't have to give up sweet foods altogether, rather, just make healthier choices.

COMPLIANT FOODS

- Foods that naturally contain sugar
- Unsweetened beverages

NON-COMPLIANT FOODS

- Foods with added sugar

- Sweetened beverages

- Sugar, honey, molasses

FOODS WITH NATURAL SUGARS

Fruits and 100 percent fruit juice are naturally sweet, but they aren't classified as having added sugar (some research shows that this is confusing to consumers).2 The exception is fruit drinks, such as most cranberry juice beverages that are a combination of fruit juices with sugar and water.

With natural sugars like those found in fruit, you may need to watch the calorie count. A glass of fruit juice may have as many calories as the same size glass of sugary soft drink. But at least the juice also has vitamins and minerals.

Unsweetened Beverages

Soda, lemonade, sweetened iced tea, and many sports drinks and energy drinks often contain added sugars. Milk has its own natural sugar (lactose). Drink plain or carbonated water, unsweetened tea or coffee, or fruit juice (in moderation). Or use a zero-calorie sweetener like stevia or sucralose.

Pastries, cookies, candy bars, syrups, jams, jellies, and pre-sweetened breakfast cereals are all obvious sources of added sugars. But other foods such as salad dressings, sauces, condiments, flavored yogurts, instant oatmeal, and fruit smoothies can also contain added sugars.

For cereal, look for brands that have less than 5 grams sugar per serving, and choose the ones with the most fiber. Or make your own oatmeal or plain unsweetened cereal and add fruits and berries. Similarly, buy plain yogurt and add fresh fruit.

In general, choose whole foods whenever you can. Processed foods tend to have added sugar, salt, and/or fat. Similarly, simple carbohydrates (such as white flour, white rice, and pasta) don't contain added sugar, but they do break down into sugar quickly in the body. So choose complex carbohydrates, like whole grains.

PROS AND CONS

Pros

- Weight loss

- Improved health

- Improved dental health

Cons

- Challenging to achieve

PROS

Weight Loss

Cutting out sugar means cutting out empty (non-nutritious) calories. Doing that should help you lose weight. And whole, nutrient-dense foods tend to be more filling, so you can eat less of them and still feel full.

Improved Health

Along with the health benefits of weight loss, a no sugar diet can help users avoid other health risks that go along with high sugar intake. For example, one research review listed three studies that showed consumption of sugar-

sweetened beverages was associated with

increased blood pressure, inflammatory markers,

total cholesterol, and visceral (belly) fat.4

Improved Dental Health

Your mom was right: Too much sugar will rot

your teeth. So a no sugar diet should help lower

your risk of dental decay.

Following a no sugar diet (or even a low sugar

diet) should offer health benefits including

weight loss. But it can be difficult to truly cut

sugar from your life.

CONS

Challenging to Achieve

Setting aside the common American taste for sugar, there is sugar hiding in many foods (some of them quite unexpected). And distinguishing added sugars from natural sugars can also be difficult. All this means that following a no sugar diet can be hard.

STARTING NO SUGAR DIET

Start gradually

Creating an eating plan you can stick to is key.

For many people, this means starting slowly.

Think of the first few weeks as a period of lower

sugar instead of no sugar. Your taste buds and palate can be "retrained" to adopt a less sugary lifestyle, and eventually you will not crave the same high-sugar foods as before.

During this time, you can still eat foods with natural sugars, like fruit, as these are packed with nutrients and fiber. As your knowledge base grows, you should begin to make small changes to your diet to decrease your intake of sugars.

You can

Try putting less sweetener in your coffee, tea, or breakfast cereal.

Swap regular soda and fruit juices for a flavored carbonated water that has no artificial sweeteners. Another option is to infuse your water with your favorite fruit.

Reach for unflavored yogurt instead of your usual full-flavor pick. Try flavoring your own plain yogurt with berries.

Be mindful of how much dried fruit you eat, as it often has added sugar on top of its higher naturally occurring sugar content. Replace dried mango and other fruits with fresh berries.

Choose whole wheat breads, pastas, and other grains with no added sugar. Read labels to make sure you're not getting added sugar in foods.

Many people deal with sugar withdrawal during the first week, so if you're feeling cranky or craving sugar, you're not alone. Making small changes like these can help ease your cravings and put you on the path to success.

Cut the obvious sources

You don't have to be a label reader to know that sugary sweets are off limits.

These include:

- breakfast pastries, like muffins and coffee cake

- baked goods, like cookies and cake

- frozen treats, like ice cream and sorbet

Note that some foods with naturally occurring sugar are often nutrient-dense, high in fiber, and can be a part of a healthy, well-balanced diet.

However, as you settle into your new routine,

you can also remove foods high in naturally

occurring sugar from your diet. This will further

train your brain to have fewer cravings.

These include:

- dried fruits, like dates and raisins

- yogurt with added fruit or other flavors

- milk

Start reading food labels

Switching to a no-sugar lifestyle often carries a

learning curve. There's hidden sugar in many, if

not most, products found on supermarket

shelves.

For example, hidden sugars can be found in:

- baked beans

- crackers

- tacos

- boxed rice

- frozen entrees

- grains, like bread, rice, and pasta

The simplest way to eliminate hidden sources of

sugar is to read the nutritional information and

ingredients list found on the food label.

Keep in mind:

- Sugar is often measured in grams on labels. Four grams is the equivalent of one teaspoon.

- Some foods, like fruit, don't come with an ingredients label. This means you'll have to look up the nutritional information online.

- Nutrition labels will soon have additional information to help you make informed decisions. The new label must list both total sugars and added sugars.

- Reading store labels can be confusing, so it may help to do some research ahead of time. There are also shopping apps, like Fooducate, that you can download right to your phone to help you check food

facts on the go.

Sugar has many sneaky aliases, and you'll need to

learn them all to completely remove it from your

diet.

A general rule of thumb is to look out for

ingredients ending in "ose" — these are usually

forms of sugar.

For example:

- glucose

- maltrose

- sucrose

- dextrose

- fructose

- lactose

In addition to clearly labeled sugars, such as malt sugar, the substance can take on many other forms.

These include:

- molasses

- agave

- syrups, such as corn, rice, malt, and maple

- fruit juice concentrate

- maltodextrin

If this sounds daunting, take heart. Once you've learned to identify sugar in all its forms, it will be easier to avoid it and stick to your plan.

Artificial sweeteners can be anywhere from 200 to 13,000 times sweeter than real sugar. This can fool your brain into thinking that you're actually eating sugar.

In the long run, these substitutes can trigger sugar cravings, making it harder for you to stick to your eating plan.

Common sugar substitutes include:

- Stevia

- Splenda

- Equal

- Sweet 'N Low

- Nutrasweet

Although they're usually marketed as a sugar replacement for cooking and baking, they're often used as ingredients in some food products.

Ingredients to watch for include:

- saccharin

- aspartame

- neotame

- sucralose

- acesulfame potassium

Often, sugar substitutes are found in products sold as no-sugar, low-sugar, or low-calorie.

Don't drink it

It's not just what you eat that matters. It's also what you drink.

Sugar can be found in:

- soda

- fruit juices

- flavored coffee

- flavored milk

- flavored tea

- hot chocolate

- tonic water

Cocktails and after-dinner liqueurs are also high in sugar. Wine, even if it's dry, contains naturally occurring sugar derived from grapes.

Opt for the unsweetened version

Many foods and drinks come in sweetened and unsweetened varieties. In most cases, the sweetened form is the default product. There usually isn't any indication that it's sweetened beyond the ingredients listing.

An "unsweetened" designation on the label is usually a sign that the item doesn't contain added sugar. However, naturally occurring sugars may still be present. Take care to read the label thoroughly before making your selection.

Removing sugar from your diet doesn't mean eliminating flavor. Look to spices, seasonings, and other natural ingredients to add some variety to your meals.

For example, drop a cinnamon stick into your cup of coffee or sprinkle the spice onto a cup of unflavored yogurt.

Vanilla is another option. The extract can add a delicious flavor to the foods you used to sweeten with sugar, and you can use the whole bean to brew iced coffee or tea.

When eliminating foods laden with natural sugar, like fruit, it's important to add other foods that can provide the same nutrients.

For example, fruit is usually high in vitamin A, vitamin C, and fiber. Vegetables can serve as an easy replacement for many fruit servings. Eat a variety of colors of vegetables to ensure you are getting the full spectrum of nutrients. Each color represents a different nutrient the body needs.

You may also wish to add a daily supplement to your routine. Talk to your doctor about your diet plan and how you can best meet your nutritional needs.

Fully eliminating natural and added sugars is not easy to do. If the thought of never eating another piece of birthday cake is too much to bear, know that total abstinence may not be necessary. The American Heart Association recommends we limit our added sugar intake to nine teaspoons for men per day and six teaspoons for women per day.

Remember, once you retrain your palate, your desire for extra sweet foods won't be as great. When adding sugar back in your diet, start with naturally occurring sugars, like in fruit. You will find these to taste sweeter, and they'll be more satisfying once you have gone through the sugar elimination process.

Think of sugar like your favorite holiday. Knowing that there's a sugary occasion to work toward may help you stick to your goals. On set occasions, sugar can be eagerly anticipated, fully savored, and then tucked away until next time.

NO SUGAR DIET COOKBOOK

RUSTIC VEGETABLE FRITTATA

Ingredients

- 1 medium sweet potato, peeled and cut into 1/4-inch slices

- 2 tablespoons water

- 7 large eggs

- 3 tablespoons fat-free milk

- 1/4 teaspoon salt

- 1/8 teaspoon pepper

- 6 center-cut bacon strips, coarsely chopped

- 1 small green pepper, chopped

- 1/2 cup chopped red onion

- 2 cups coarsely chopped fresh kale

Directions

- Preheat oven to 375°. Place sweet potato and water in a microwave-safe bowl; microwave, covered, on high until potato is just tender, 5-6 minutes; drain.

- Meanwhile, whisk together eggs, milk, salt and pepper. In a 10-in. oven-safe skillet, cook bacon over medium heat until crisp, stirring occasionally. Using a slotted spoon, remove bacon to paper towels. Remove all but 1 tablespoon drippings from pan.

- In drippings, saute green pepper, onion and kale over medium heat until tender, 4-5 minutes. Reduce heat to low. Stir in egg mixture; add potato and bacon. Cook until eggs are partially set, 1-2 minutes.

- Transfer to oven; bake until eggs are set, 5-7 minutes. Cut into wedges.

- Test Kitchen tips

- Center-cut bacon has more meat and less fat per strip. Regular bacon can be used, too.

- Finishing the frittata in the oven instead of on the stovetop will keep the bottom from getting too dark.

- Frittatas can also be served cold, which makes them easy to pack for lunch or a picnic.

ROASTED BUTTERNUT LINGUINE

Ingredients

- 4 cups cubed peeled butternut squash

- 1 medium red onion, chopped

- 3 tablespoons olive oil

- 1/4 teaspoon crushed red pepper flakes

- 1/2 pound uncooked linguine

- 2 cups julienned Swiss chard

- 1 tablespoon minced fresh sage

- 1/2 teaspoon salt

- 1/4 teaspoon pepper

Directions

- Preheat oven to 350°. Place the squash

  and onion in a 15x10x1-in. baking pan

coated with cooking spray. Combine the

oil and pepper flakes; drizzle over

vegetables and toss to coat.

- Bake, uncovered, 45-50 minutes or until

tender, stirring occasionally.

- Meanwhile, cook linguine according to

package directions; drain and place in a

large bowl. Add squash mixture, Swiss

chard, sage, salt and pepper; toss to

combine.

ROAST PORK WITH APPLES & ONIONS

Ingredients

- 1 boneless pork loin roast (2 pounds)

- 1/4 teaspoon salt

- 1/4 teaspoon pepper

- 1 tablespoon olive oil

- 3 large Golden Delicious apples, cut into

  1-inch wedges

- 2 large onions, cut into 3/4-inch wedges

- 5 garlic cloves, peeled

- 1 tablespoon minced fresh rosemary or 1

  teaspoon dried rosemary, crushed

Directions

- Preheat oven to 350°. Sprinkle roast with

  salt and pepper. In a large nonstick skillet,

  heat oil over medium heat; brown roast

  on all sides. Transfer to a roasting pan

  coated with cooking spray. Place apples,

onions and garlic around roast; sprinkle with rosemary.

- Roast until a thermometer inserted in pork reads 145°, 45-55 minutes, turning apples, onion and garlic once. Remove from oven; tent with foil. Let stand 10 minutes before slicing roast. Serve with apple mixture.

WHAT'S IN THE FRIDGE FRITTATA

Ingredients

- 6 large eggs

- 1/3 cup chopped onion

- 1/3 cup chopped sweet red pepper

- 1/3 cup chopped fresh mushrooms

- 1 tablespoon olive oil

- 1 can (6 ounces) lump crabmeat, drained

- 1/4 cup shredded Swiss cheese

- 1 tablespoon minced fresh parsley,
  optional

Directions

- In a small bowl, whisk eggs; set aside. In
  an 8-in. ovenproof skillet, saute the onion,
  pepper and mushrooms in oil until tender.
  Reduce heat; sprinkle with crab. Top with
  eggs. Cover and cook until nearly set, 5-7
  minutes.

- Uncover skillet; sprinkle with cheese and,
  if desired, parsley. Broil 3-4 in. from the

heat until eggs are completely set, 2-3
minutes. Let stand for 5 minutes. Cut into
wedges.

AVOCADO & ARTICHOKE PASTA SALAD

Ingredients

- 2 cups uncooked gemelli or spiral pasta

- 1 can (14 ounces) water-packed artichoke
  hearts, drained and coarsely chopped

- 2 plum tomatoes, seeded and chopped

- 1 medium ripe avocado, peeled and
  cubed

- 1/4 cup grated Romano cheese

DRESSING:

- 1/4 cup canola oil

- 2 tablespoons lime juice

- 1 tablespoon minced fresh cilantro

- 1-1/2 teaspoons grated lime zest

- 1/2 teaspoon kosher salt

- 1/2 teaspoon freshly ground pepper

Directions

- Cook pasta according to package

  directions. Drain; rinse with cold water.

- In a large bowl, combine pasta, artichoke

  hearts, tomatoes, avocado and cheese. In

  a small bowl, whisk dressing ingredients.

  Pour over pasta mixture; toss gently to

  combine. Refrigerate, covered, until

  serving.

DEVILED CHICKEN

Ingredients

- 6 chicken leg quarters

- 1/4 cup butter, melted

- 1 tablespoon lemon juice

- 1 tablespoon prepared mustard

- 1 teaspoon salt

- 1 teaspoon paprika

- 1/4 teaspoon pepper

Directions

- Preheat oven to 375°. Place chicken in a 15x10x1-in. baking pan. In a small bowl, combine remaining ingredients. Pour over chicken.

- Bake, uncovered, 50-60 minutes or until a thermometer reads 170°-175°, basting occasionally with pan juices.

APPLE CINNAMON OVERNIGHT OATS

ingredients

- 1/2 cup old-fashioned oats
- 1/2 medium Gala or Honeycrisp apple, chopped
- 1 tablespoon raisins
- 1 cup 2% milk
- 1/4 teaspoon ground cinnamon

- Dash salt

- Toasted, chopped nuts, optional

Directions

- In a small container or Mason jar, combine all ingredients. Seal; refrigerate overnight. Makes 1 serving.

MEDITERRANEAN COBB SALAD

Ingredients

- 1 package (6 ounces) falafel mix

- 1/2 cup sour cream or plain yogurt

- 1/4 cup chopped seeded peeled cucumber

- 1/4 cup 2% milk

- 1 teaspoon minced fresh parsley

- 1/4 teaspoon salt

- 4 cups torn romaine

- 4 cups fresh baby spinach

- 3 hard-boiled large eggs, chopped

- 2 medium tomatoes, seeded and finely

  chopped

- 1 medium ripe avocado, peeled and finely

  chopped

- 3/4 cup crumbled feta cheese

- 8 bacon strips, cooked and crumbled

- 1/2 cup pitted Greek olives, finely

  chopped

Directions

- Prepare and cook falafel according to package directions. When cool enough to handle, crumble or coarsely chop falafel.

- In a small bowl, mix sour cream, cucumber, milk, parsley and salt. In a large bowl, combine romaine and spinach; transfer to a platter. Arrange crumbled falafel and remaining ingredients over greens. Drizzle with dressing.

WHITE CHEDDAR MAC & CHEESE

Ingredients

- 1 package (16 ounces) small pasta shells
- 1/2 cup butter, cubed

- 1/2 cup all-purpose flour

- 1/2 teaspoon onion powder

- 1/2 teaspoon ground chipotle pepper

- 1/2 teaspoon pepper

- 1/4 teaspoon salt

- 4 cups 2% milk

- 2 cups shredded sharp white cheddar cheese

- 2 cups shredded Manchego or additional white cheddar cheese

Directions

- In a 6-qt. stockpot, cook pasta according to package directions. Drain; return to pot.

- Meanwhile, in a large saucepan, melt butter over medium heat. Stir in flour and seasonings until smooth; gradually whisk in milk. Bring to a boil, stirring constantly; cook and stir until thickened, 6-8 minutes. Remove from heat; stir in cheeses until melted. Add to pasta; toss to coat.

VERY VEGGIE FRITTATA

Ingredients

- 5 large eggs
- 1/4 cup sour cream
- 1/4 teaspoon salt
- 1/8 teaspoon pepper

- 1 cup shredded cheddar cheese, divided

- 2 green onions, chopped

- 1 cup chopped fresh mushrooms

- 1/2 cup each chopped sweet red, yellow

  and green pepper

- 1/4 cup chopped onion

- 1 tablespoon butter

- Hot pepper sauce, optional

Directions

- In a large bowl, whisk the eggs, sour

  cream, salt and pepper. Stir in 3/4 cup

  cheese and green onions; set aside. In a 9-

  in. ovenproof skillet, saute the

  mushrooms, sweet peppers and onion in

  butter until tender. Reduce heat; top with

egg mixture. Cover and cook for 4-6 minutes or until nearly set.

- Uncover skillet; sprinkle with remaining cheese. Broil 3-4 in. from the heat for 2-3 minutes or until eggs are completely set. Let stand for 5 minutes. Cut into wedges. Serve with pepper sauce, if desired.

GARLIC LEMON SHRIMP

Ingredients

- 2 tablespoons olive oil

- 1 pound uncooked shrimp (26-30 per pound), peeled and deveined

- 3 garlic cloves, thinly sliced

- 1 tablespoon lemon juice

- 1 teaspoon ground cumin

- 1/4 teaspoon salt

- 2 tablespoons minced fresh parsley

- Hot cooked pasta or rice

Directions

- In a large skillet, heat oil over medium-high heat; saute shrimp 3 minutes. Add garlic, lemon juice, cumin and salt; cook and stir until shrimp turn pink. Stir in parsley. Serve with pasta.

- Health Tip: Cooking the shrimp in olive oil instead of butter saves about 3 grams of saturated fat per serving.

QUICK CHICKEN PICCATA

Ingredients

- 1/4 cup all-purpose flour

- 1/2 teaspoon salt

- 1/2 teaspoon pepper

- 4 boneless skinless chicken breast halves

  (4 ounces each)

- 1/4 cup butter, cubed

- 1/4 cup white wine or chicken broth

- 1 tablespoon lemon juice

- Minced fresh parsley, optional

Directions

- In a shallow bowl, mix flour, salt and pepper. Pound chicken breasts with a meat mallet to 1/2-in. thickness. Dip chicken in flour mixture to coat both sides; shake off excess.

- In a large skillet, heat butter over medium heat. Brown chicken on both sides. Add wine; bring to a boil. Reduce heat; simmer, uncovered, until chicken is no longer pink, 12-15 minutes. Drizzle with lemon juice. If desired, sprinkle with parsley.

- Test Kitchen Tips

- Unless otherwise specified, Taste of Home recipes are tested with lightly salted butter. Unsalted, or sweet, butter is sometimes used to achieve a buttery flavor, such as in shortbread cookies or buttercream frosting. In these recipes, added salt would detract from the buttery taste desired.

- Lemon juice in this zesty marinade is an acid, which breaks down the tough proteins in the pork and helps to tenderize it.

ZUCCHINI FRITTATA

Ingredients

- 3 large eggs

- 1/4 teaspoon salt

- 1 teaspoon canola oil

- 1/2 cup chopped onion

- 1 cup coarsely shredded zucchini

- 1/2 cup shredded Swiss cheese

- Coarsely ground pepper, optional

Directions

- Preheat oven to 350°. Whisk together

  eggs and salt.

- In an 8-in. ovenproof skillet coated with

  cooking spray, heat oil over medium heat;

  saute onion and zucchini until onion is

  crisp-tender. Pour in egg mixture; cook

  until almost set, 5-6 minutes. Sprinkle

  with cheese.

- Bake, uncovered, until cheese is melted, 4-5 minutes. If desired, sprinkle with pepper.

FARMERS MARKET ORZO SALAD

Ingredients

- 1 package (16 ounces) orzo pasta

- 2 small yellow summer squash, halved lengthwise

- 1 medium zucchini, halved lengthwise

- 1 medium red onion, quartered

- 8 tablespoons olive oil, divided

- 1/2 teaspoon salt, divided

- 1/4 teaspoon pepper, divided

- 3 tablespoons lemon juice

- 8 ounces smoked mozzarella cheese, cut
  into 1/4-inch cubes

- 1-1/2 cups grape tomatoes, halved
  lengthwise

- 1/2 cup chopped fresh basil

- 1/2 cup pine nuts, toasted

Directions

- Cook orzo according to package
  directions; drain. Brush yellow squash,
  zucchini and onion with 2 tablespoons oil;
  sprinkle with 1/4 teaspoon salt and 1/8
  teaspoon pepper. Grill vegetables,
  covered, over medium heat or broil 4 in.
  from heat 10-12 minutes or until lightly

charred and tender, turning once. Cool slightly. Cut into 1-in. pieces.

- In a small bowl, whisk lemon juice and remaining oil until blended. In a large bowl, combine orzo, grilled vegetables, mozzarella, tomatoes, basil and remaining salt and pepper. Add dressing; toss to coat. Sprinkle with pine nuts.

CUMIN-CHILI SPICED FLANK STEAK

Ingredients

- 2 small sweet red peppers, cut into 2-inch strips

- 1 small sweet yellow pepper, cut into 2-inch strips

- 2 cups grape tomatoes

- 1 small onion, cut into 1/2-inch wedges

- 2 jalapeno peppers, halved and seeded

- 2 tablespoons olive oil, divided

- 3/4 teaspoon salt, divided

- 3/4 teaspoon pepper, divided

- 2 teaspoons ground cumin

- 1 teaspoon chili powder

- 1 beef flank steak (1-1/2 pounds)

- 2 to 3 teaspoons lime juice

- Hot cooked couscous

- Lime wedges

Directions

- Preheat broiler. Place the first 5
  ingredients in a greased 15x10x1-in.
  baking pan. Toss with 1 tablespoon oil,
  1/4 teaspoon salt and 1/4 teaspoon
  pepper. Broil 4 in. from heat 10-12
  minutes or until vegetables are tender
  and begin to char, turning once.

- Meanwhile, mix salt, pepper, cumin, chili
  powder and the remaining oil; rub over
  both sides of steak. Grill, covered, over
  medium heat or broil 4 in. from heat 6-9
  minutes on each side or until meat
  reaches desired doneness (for medium-
  rare, a thermometer should read 135°;

medium, 140°; medium-well, 145°). Let stand 5 minutes.

- For salsa, chop broiled onion and jalapenos; place in a small bowl. Stir in tomatoes and lime juice. Thinly slice steak across the grain; serve with salsa, broiled peppers, couscous and lime wedges.

SOUTHWEST TORTILLA SCRAMBLE

Ingredients

- 4 large egg whites

- 2 large eggs

- 1/4 teaspoon pepper

- 2 corn tortillas (6 inches), halved and cut into strips

- 1/4 cup chopped fresh spinach

- 2 tablespoons shredded reduced-fat cheddar cheese

- 1/4 cup salsa

Directions

- In a large bowl, whisk egg whites, eggs and pepper. Stir in tortillas, spinach and cheese.

- Heat a large skillet coated with cooking spray over medium heat. Pour in egg mixture; cook and stir until eggs are thickened and no liquid egg remains. Top with salsa.

FRESH CORN AND TOMATO FETTUCCINI

Ingredients

- 8 ounces uncooked whole wheat fettuccine

- 2 medium ears sweet corn, husked

- 2 teaspoons plus 2 tablespoons olive oil, divided

- 1/2 cup chopped sweet red pepper

- 4 green onions, chopped

- 2 medium tomatoes, chopped

- 1/2 teaspoon salt

- 1/2 teaspoon pepper

- 1 cup crumbled feta cheese

- 2 tablespoons minced fresh parsley

Directions

- In a Dutch oven, cook fettuccine according to package directions, adding corn during the last 8 minutes of cooking.

- Meanwhile, in a small skillet, heat 2 teaspoons oil over medium-high heat. Add red pepper and green onions; cook and stir until tender.

- Drain pasta and corn; transfer pasta to a large bowl. Cool corn slightly; cut corn from cob and add to pasta. Add tomatoes, salt, pepper, remaining oil and the pepper mixture; toss to combine. Sprinkle with cheese and parsley.

Ingredients

- 2 pounds red potatoes (about 6 medium), cut into 3/4-inch pieces

- 1 large onion, coarsely chopped

- 2 tablespoons olive oil

- 3 garlic cloves, minced

- 1-1/4 teaspoons salt, divided

- 1 teaspoon dried rosemary, crushed, divided

- 3/4 teaspoon pepper, divided

- 1/2 teaspoon paprika

- 6 bone-in chicken thighs (about 2-1/4 pounds), skin removed

- 6 cups fresh baby spinach (about 6 ounces)

Directions

- Preheat oven to 425°. In a large bowl, combine potatoes, onion, oil, garlic, 3/4 teaspoon salt, 1/2 teaspoon rosemary and 1/2 teaspoon pepper; toss to coat. Transfer to a 15x10x1-in. baking pan coated with cooking spray.

- In a small bowl, mix paprika and the remaining salt, rosemary and pepper. Sprinkle chicken with paprika mixture; arrange over vegetables. Roast until a thermometer inserted in chicken reads 170°-175° and vegetables are just tender, 35-40 minutes.

- Remove chicken to a serving platter; keep warm. Top vegetables with spinach. Roast until vegetables are tender and spinach is wilted, 8-10 minutes longer. Stir vegetables to combine; serve with chicken.

Test Kitchen Tips

- Prepare your sheet-pan meal the night before and just pop it into the preheated oven to bake. This helps to deeply flavor the chicken, a win-win!

- If you want a richer dish, use skin-on chicken, and if you want a lighter dish, use bone-in chicken breasts. Be sure to cook bone-in breasts just to 165-170 degrees, since leaner meat can become dry at higher temperatures.

- Keep an eye out for the most common sheet pan dinner mistakes.

TURKEY BREAKFAST SAUSAGE

Ingredients

- 1 pound lean ground turkey

- 3/4 teaspoon salt

- 1/2 teaspoon rubbed sage

- 1/2 teaspoon pepper

- 1/4 teaspoon ground ginger

Directions

- Crumble turkey into a large bowl. Add the salt, sage, pepper and ginger. Shape into eight 2-in. patties.

- In a greased cast-iron or other heavy skillet, cook patties over medium heat until a thermometer reads 165° and juices run clear, 4-6 minutes on each side.

GRILLED SOUTHWESTERN STEAK SALAD

Ingredients

- 1 beef top sirloin steak (1 inch thick and

  3/4 pound)

- 1/4 teaspoon salt

- 1/4 teaspoon ground cumin

- 1/4 teaspoon pepper

- 3 poblano peppers, halved and seeded

- 2 large ears sweet corn, husks removed

- 1 large sweet onion, cut into 1/2-inch

  rings

- 1 tablespoon olive oil

- 2 cups uncooked multigrain bow tie pasta

- 2 large tomatoes

DRESSING:

- 1/4 cup lime juice

- 1 tablespoon olive oil

- 1/4 teaspoon salt

- 1/4 teaspoon ground cumin

- 1/4 teaspoon pepper

- 1/3 cup chopped fresh cilantro

Directions

- Rub steak with salt, cumin and pepper.
  Brush poblano peppers, corn and onion
  with oil. Grill steak, covered, over medium
  heat or broil 4 in. from heat 6-8 minutes
  on each side or until meat reaches desired
  doneness (for medium-rare, a
  thermometer should read 135°; medium,
  140°; medium-well, 145°). Grill

vegetables, covered, 8-10 minutes or until

crisp-tender, turning occasionally.

- Cook pasta according to package

  directions. Meanwhile, cut corn from cob;

  coarsely chop peppers, onion and

  tomatoes. Transfer vegetables to a large

  bowl. In a small bowl, whisk lime juice, oil,

  salt, cumin and pepper until blended; stir

  in cilantro.

- Drain pasta; add to vegetable mixture.

  Drizzle with dressing; toss to coat. Cut

  steak into thin slices; add to salad.

GRILLED BASIL CHICKEN AND TOMATOES

Ingredients

- 3/4 cup balsamic vinegar

- 1/4 cup tightly packed fresh basil leaves

- 2 tablespoons olive oil

- 1 garlic clove, minced

- 1/2 teaspoon salt

- 8 plum tomatoes

- 4 boneless skinless chicken breast halves

  (4 ounces each)

Directions

- For marinade, place first five ingredients

  in a blender. Cut four tomatoes into

  quarters and add to blender; cover and

  process until blended. Halve remaining

  tomatoes for grilling.

- In a bowl, combine chicken and 2/3 cup marinade; refrigerate, covered, 1 hour, turning occasionally. Reserve remaining marinade for serving.

- Place chicken on an oiled grill rack over medium heat; discard marinade remaining in bowl. Grill chicken, covered, until a thermometer reads 165°, 4-6 minutes per side. Grill tomatoes, covered, over medium heat until lightly browned, 2-4 minutes per side. Serve chicken and tomatoes with reserved marinade.rilled Basil Chicken and Tomatoes

CONCLUSION

Going completely sugar-free isn't for everyone.

However, limiting sugar is something most

anyone can do, even if for a short period of time.

You may wish to alternate your no-sugar diet

with a low-sugar diet from week to week. You

could also try avoiding refined sugars but

reintroducing naturally occurring sugars, like in

fruits, back into your diet.

No matter how you reduce your sugar intake,

making a concerted effort to do so is likely to

have a positive impact. It can help your skin clear

up, increase your energy levels, and reduce

excess weight you've been carrying. These health

benefits will only increase over the long-term.